PRACTICE PEARLS

A COMPREHENSIVE GUIDE ON THE TRANSITION FROM NURSE TO PROVIDER

Shelita S Carr MSN APRN FNP-C CCRN

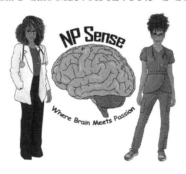

DEDICATION

This book is dedicated to every individual that has a dream or goal but is unsure of how to accomplish it. I dedicate this book to anyone who is simply unsure if you can fit anymore in your already cramped life. I sat on my goal of writing this book for over five years because I could not find the time to fit it in my work schedule (as I had to work, it was not an option). I sat on my goal to write this book because I did not know how to start. I sat on my goal because I did not know how to finish. Yet, one day, this little voice in my head said, "The time is now. Write your book!"
I believe that was the Holy Spirit speaking to me, teaching me how to find the time and putting the right interactions together. I believe God was saying, "This is your season. Conquer your goals." And that is what I did. So, for anyone not knowing how to accomplish or conquer their dreams, I dedicate this book to you. I am a living testimony that if I can write this book and conquer my goals, so can you. I dedicate my completed goal (this book) to you. Never give up.
Conquer your dreams.
.

CONTENTS

TESTIMONIALS

"I was blessed to have met Shelita during my first year in practice. She has educated, supported, and empowered me through my own transition into the role of the provider. No educational program [fully] prepares you for the transition from nurse to provider, and there is none better suited to guide others in finding their own path into the profession than Shelita. She is not only knowledgeable in her specialty; she is loved by her patients, respected in her community, and admired by her colleagues."
– Lily, APRN FNP-C

"Shelita Carr is someone I aspire to be as a Nurse Practitioner. She takes her craft seriously, and her patients love and respect her. Her knowledge base is unmatched, as she is able to assess, diagnose, and treat using an evidence-based practice. She is respected by all her peers as well as the students she selflessly precepts throughout the year. She willingly offers her knowledge to others, and this book is her gift to us all."
– Rasheeda Plessy, BSN, RN

"Mrs. Carr is a walking medical dictionary. She is highly respected by medical professionals in our region and is a ray of sunshine to everybody she comes in contact with. The knowledge I've received from her

throughout the years has been invaluable to me. I am excited to learn more knowledge and pearls that will be shared in this book and apply it to my practice."
– Mikshira Mosley, MSN, APRN, FNP-C

"To know Shelita is to know strength. To be in her presence is to know compassion. Shelita Carr is an inspirational presence to the profession of nursing. Her wealth of knowledge and willingness to teach others are stellar. She uses her advanced studies in nursing as a foundation or a blueprint, if you will, to present the best plan for her patients. She not only elevates you but pours priceless gems of knowledge into those who are willing and open to receive. God bless your endeavors; we are blessed to have you in the nursing profession."
– Kimberly Dickerson, MSN, RN

"As a friend of many years, I have watched Shelita grow into this super beautiful butterfly. You have been a wealth of knowledge for everyone, including me. You are known to be ingenious, wise, nimble, and that "go-to person" for academic advice. Your educational growth has fostered several nurses thus far, and this book will give a positive pathway of edification and advancement to others."
– Tonyell Woodridge, MSN, APRN, FNP-C

"Who better to write a book about any and everything pertaining to the Nurse Practitioner other than Shelita Carr? She is the epitome of nursing, the best to ever do it. I cannot think of a more perfect person to give insight on what it is and takes to function as an NP in today's NP world. She is knowledgeable, intuitive, positive, honest, caring, and the most passionate NP you will find today. She eats and breathes nursing daily. She honestly does not know how to cut it off. Shelita is the reason I went back to school. If you have ever had a chance to meet her, you know what I mean when I say, "Motivational!" Just one conversation

with her will have you wanting to do more. She has that impact on people. There are plenty of people she has influenced in a very positive way. Shelita is the [epitome] of a goal setter/go-getter! Whatever she sets her mind to, it's done! She's one of a kind, an intelligent black Queen, [and] a genius in my eyes. Purchase her book. Read her book. Devour her book. She is going to give you the tools needed to transition from RN to NP with ease. This book will be informative, relatable, and reliable. I can't wait for her book signings, for [you all] to get a glimpse of what I've had the privilege of experiencing for the last twenty-plus years [I've known her]. Just one meeting, your life will forever be changed… I guarantee it!"
– Avis Elayne Gay, CRT

"As I think back over [my] twenty-five years of nursing experience, I often reflect on students/colleagues who have had an impact on my life. I have mentored many students, but Shelita stands out as a practitioner as well as a person. If I had to describe her in two words, it would be exceptional and compassionate. Her ability, knowledge base, and skills are exceptional. But more importantly, combined with all the skills and abilities, she has a heart. I know you thought I was mentoring you, but the entire time, you were motivating and inspiring me. Thank you, Shelita, for allowing me to be a part of your professional journey. You are truly a great asset to the healthcare profession."
– Dr. Rhonda Maberry

"Shelita has been a mentor to me for several years. She is the type of medical professional every patient needs at their bedside. Her skill set and knowledge base are accompanied by a drive to deliver care that promotes the highest possible outcomes. She has educated, inspired, and empowered me to become a stronger nurse."
– Stephanie Bisesi, RN

"I would like to thank Shelita Carr for the knowledge, inspiration, guidance, and professionalism in which she has inculcated in me. Thanks for being such a great prodigy and mentor. Also, thanks for sharing your gift and time with me and others. I know with all certainty this book will dispense the expertise that [will] embrace [its readers]."
– Janel Isom, APRN, FNP-C

"Shelita has an undeniable commitment to every aspect of quality health care. She has provided insurmountable guidance and leadership to fellow NPs. [This book], written by Mrs. Carr, will become a standard textbook."
– Ahsaki George–Scharpon, APRN, FNP-C

"Shelita is a smart, hardworking, and compassionate person. I have learned so much with her during our time together. She is an advocate for her patients and loves what she does. I am so proud of her accomplishments."
– Dominiece Lacroix, APRN, FNP-C

"I have known Shelita for nearly twenty years, starting as a bedside nurse, then becoming a nurse manager, and finally a mid-level provider. During that time, she has consistently performed very well in all her roles. And now, with her years of experience as a mid-level [provider], her skill set is simply excellent."
– Demetrix P Tolliver, FACHE

"Mrs. Carr has exhibited persistent professional growth and knowledge for [the] many years I have been fortunate enough to know her. Not only has she continued to teach and groom me, but she also shows a great desire to enhance the growth of the community and peers around her. I am excited for the knowledge that will be shared in this project because I know it is of great value and expertise from one of the most highly

respected medical professionals in the region."
– Shemika Bradford, APRN, FNP-C

"[Shelita Carr is a] dynamic nurse and mentor. I often ask God to reveal my gift so that I might follow His plan before leaving this earth. What He has shown me was your gift that He bestowed upon you [and] I have been blessed to have been touched by you and your journey. I'm not sure how we even became friends; it just happened. You have been my inspiration, my mentor, and my champion. Some of your struggles, I have witnessed, [but] your accomplishments have been beyond belief. Your success story will forever be a part of me. Know that you will go far beyond what you have imagined. Ecclesiastes 3:1 [says], 'There is a season (at a time appointed) for everything and a time for every delight and event or purpose under heaven.' It's your season, so shine bright like the diamond you are."
– Johnether Smith, APRN, FNP-C

"I don't know where to start when speaking of Shelita. I believe her gift is love. Shelita puts love into everything she says and does. Shelita is the reason I'm a nurse. She made being a nurse the coolest thing in the world. She made becoming a nurse look so easy [but] it wasn't. [However], here I am, killing it … I mean, here I am saving the world! Shelita, you are the epitome of nursing, our very own Florence Nightingale. You are a born leader. God designed you perfectly in His image. Yes, you are perfect. I see you teaching in the classroom, performing brain surgery, transplanting a heart, you name it! I believe you can do it. You are [the definition of] black girl magic, and I cannot wait to see what hospital you will be the CEO of. Love you, sister and friend. You rock!"
– Rachelle Stone, RN, BSN

"Shelita Carr, I'm beyond amazed. Your intelligence, grace, and

humbleness are gleaming through your words of encouragement. I feel this book is just what a novel APRN [like] myself needs. You are so knowledgeable [and] I can't wait to see what else you have to offer."
– Cabrina Ridley, RN, FNP student

ACKNOWLEDGMENTS

A lot of incredibly special people helped me turn this book into a reality. First and foremost, I give God all the praises and thanks for the goals he continually allows me to achieve. Without Him, I am nothing, and this book would never be possible. Secondly, I want to thank my husband, Ronald Carr Jr., for his patience and understanding during the nights I should have spent with him but instead spent at the computer working on yet another project that was dear to me. Thank you so much for believing in me and allowing me to be me without gripe or irritation. Thank you for the constant reminders, assuring me I could complete this project while working the hours I do. Your support will never be forgotten.

Thanks to my family and friends for all the support provided. I want to give a special thanks to Avis Gay, my best friend, for being my biggest cheerleader. Lastly, I want to give a huge thanks to Shemika Bradford, APRN, FNP-C, Cabrina Ridley, RN, FNP student, and Melanie Redmond (mentor) for all the feedback and great information on revisions. Thanks for helping my dream become a reality.

PREFACE

Welcome to the fantastic world of the healthcare provider. Take a deep breath and be confident knowing you have mastered the basics in your program. You are ready!

There are six main objectives this comprehensive guide aims to teach: 1) how to approach the new world of provider when choosing your workplace interests, 2) how to avoid the pitfalls of unsafe work conditions while remaining flexible, 3) how to market yourself while maintaining realistic expectations, 4) how to communicate with your new physician colleagues as a peer and not a subordinate, 5) how to safely manage your patient as a new provider, and most importantly, 6) how to confidently transition from the role of bedside nurse to provider.

This information is necessary to maintain workplace satisfaction, happiness, and success. As you move forward on your journey, keep in mind that health is wealth, and without happiness, your career and hard work are null. So please relax, get informed, and go get the job that is meant for you! Disclaimer: Please keep in mind that the material in this book is exclusively subjective and reflective of my experiences as a novel APRN expanding into an experienced APRN, as well as those of my colleagues, who have recounted jarringly similar experiences. Though these experiences may be common, they are not all-inclusive.

ABBREVIATIONS

ADD: Attention Deficit Disorder
ADHD: Attention Deficit Hyperactive Disorder
APRN: Advanced Practice Registered Nurse
BP: Blood Pressure
CNA: Certified Nursing Assistant
CCRN: A registered service mark and a brand name. It does not mean "Critical Care Registered Nurse," as the American Association of Critical-Care Nurses cannot guarantee that a certificant is a registered nurse. This is an issue between the nurse and their state.
CEO: Chief Executive Officer
CEU: Continuing Education Unit
CHADS: An acronym for the **C**ongestive heart failure, **H**ypertension, **A**ge, **D**iabetes mellitus, and **S**troke/TIA/or Systemic Embolic process, which is a scoring system utilized to determine the potential for stroke with atrial fibrillation.
CPA: Collaborative Practice Agreement
CT: Computed Tomography
DEA: Drug Enforcement Administration
ED: Emergency Department
ER: Emergency Room

ESRD: End-Stage Renal Disease
FNP: Family Nurse Practitioner
HD: Hemodialysis
HPI: History of Present Illness
HTN: Hypertension
I&D: Incision and Drainage
ICU: Intensive Care Unit
IPR: Inpatient Rehab
LPN: Licensed Practical Nurse
LTAC: Long-Term Acute Care
MA: Medical Assistant
MD: Doctor of Medicine
NH: Nursing Home
NP: Nurse Practitioner
PMR: Polymyalgia Rheumatica
RN: Registered Nurse
SLE: Systemic Lupus Erythematosus
SNF: Skilled Nursing Facility
TIMI: An acronym for **T**hrombolysis **i**n **M**yocardial and **I**nfarction, which is a score used to determine the potential for an ischemic event or the mortality risk associated with non-ST segment elevation myocardial infarction (NSTEMI for short) or unstable angina.

INTRODUCTION

Hi, my name is Shelita Carr. For the last seven years, I have been a master's prepared, actively practicing advanced practice registered nurse (APRN). My area of expertise is primarily hospital medicine, which encompasses all phases of care (medical, surgical, telemetry, and some intensive care). I also have a small clinic where I practice for half of the day after completing my hospital rounds. If that does not indicate how eventful my life is, allow me to add that I am married with five adult children and four adult stepchildren. (I know, blended families are so much fun. And yes, I have been busy in life!)

I initially started my career as a medical assistant in 1993. I then went on to become a licensed practical nurse in 1996, which was followed by my graduation as a registered nurse with an associate degree in 2002. In 2011, I attained my bachelor of science in nursing. I then decided to enter into the APRN program, keeping in mind that I was getting older and needed a solid retirement plan. When deciding what to do next, I could not see myself *not* contributing to the world of nursing; patient care seemed to be my gift. I was good at it and understood pathophysiology pretty well.

At this phase in my life, my kids were entering college, and medical school was not financially feasible or realistic for me. I decided to dedicate the next phase of my nursing career to the community by attaining a degree that would afford me the capabilities to provide sound education, diagnosis, and treatment to patients. The field of medicine, along with the edge of my nursing experience, seemed logical, so I decided to attend nurse practitioner school. In 2013, I graduated from Loyola University of New Orleans with a concentration in family medicine and completed boards two months thereafter with the American Academy of Nurse Practitioners (AANP). I am incredibly grateful for the advanced practice foundation that program provided me.

My educational time span was perfect for me because it took place in multiple phases due to the demands and necessities of working while caring for multiple kids (some periods of time as a single parent). I like to say I am a "Jackie" of all trades because my educational background has afforded me many experiences, which have all molded me into who I am today. It has also provided me with various personal and professional contacts, many of whom I now consider friends.

I chose to write this book because it is my personal belief that being an exceptionally skilled clinical registered nurse with a sound educational NP background is a blueprint for a smooth transition in the workforce of advanced practice nursing. I did not think during *any* phase of my program that I would practice with the feelings of being a "new nurse" again, especially after seventeen years of active, uninterrupted nursing experience in several aspects of health care. Though the program adequately prepared me to perform at the peak of my ability, it failed to emotionally prepare me for the transition from nurse to provider. They really are two different worlds coexisting! If not prepared both educationally and emotionally, novel APRNs can fall prey to several occurrences, including the inability to market themselves confidently, unknowingly working with physicians who dictate practice guidelines without knowledge of state restraints (most private-based positions), and a lack of overall provider confidence due to feelings of inadequacy (which is a normal phase of the novel APRN).

My goal is to provide you with a sense of what is normal during this new phase of your exciting career. If I can instill confidence in the novel APRN and make sure they know what they're experiencing is a normal part of the growing process, I have succeeded. I want to assist you in understanding and experiencing everything because while the APRN's role is fun, exhilarating, and powerful, it is also tremendously serious.

Thank you for purchasing this guide that was made explicitly for us as nurses, nursing students with a desire for advancement into the world of the APRN, and novel or seasoned advanced practice providers. Enjoy a glimpse into your new or upcoming role.

1

WELCOME TO THE WORLD OF
THE PROVIDER

Congratulations on deciding to become an advanced practice registered nurse (APRN). Whether you are a student, in the early introduction phase, or a novel nurse practitioner who has landed employment, there are vast differences in your new role when compared to that of a registered nurse. If you are not careful in your decision-making and employment choice, you can easily regret your decision as a new provider. The role of the provider is unmatched and has many positive moments; however, like any other career, it comes with its negative moments as well.

This book aims to prevent the burnout some novel APRNs face due to poor decision-making. Upon the completion of this guide, you will be able to make a more informed decision on how to proceed down the many avenues afforded to the advanced practice provider.

Please keep in mind that the nurse practitioner employment process is quite different from that of the registered nurse. I implore you to have an idea of what specialty or role you are most interested in and start looking early. Colleagues, take heed; the journey from graduation to employment is *slow*. Many nurse practitioners graduate and work as registered nurses because the timeline of application, interview, collaborative agreements, insurance attainment, and credentialing is roughly three to six months long. Know what you want and start *early*, preferably in your last semester as a nurse practitioner. Also keep in mind that most quick-hiring processes usually do not protect you as the provider and are more than likely initiated by desperate employers. These employers need you quicker for a reason and are usually willing to take shortcuts to push you into the workforce early.

It is my experience, along with many colleagues I have spoken with, that any job that pushes a novel APRN into the workforce quickly is usually not protecting them. In this scenario, the novel APRN will quickly realize they may not be a good fit and quit, thus creating a revolving door for employers that fit into this category. These quick-to-hire employers are also likely trying to take advantage of the valuable pearls you may be unaware of to maintain your license, such as scope of practice, prescribing rules, and resourcing.

2
CORPORATE VS. PRIVATE WORLD: THE PROS AND CONS

I was fortunate as a newly licensed APRN to land a job in corporate America. There were many strong positives that encompassed working in this sector. I seemed to be married to the corporate workplace, but my honeymoon ended within a few years, and nothing in my APRN program prepared me for the gradual eye-opening cons my APRN colleagues and I personally experienced. These experiences quickly contributed to my feelings of workplace despair. I soon divorced that job to embark on a journey in the private sector. Again, I was married to the private workforce, and within years, I became aware of situations and predicaments that made me reconsider my place in that sector. I quickly learned I had to pick my battles and choose the job that was best for my circumstances, whether it was in the private or corporate sector.

I have always known that the grass is not greener on the other side; however, what these disparities in the private and corporate sector have taught me is that *no* job is perfect. All working sectors come with pros and cons. As an APRN who has worked in both private and corporate sectors, it is essential to delineate the two so you may have a clear understanding of both variations. This chapter was designed to hopefully spare the fellow APRN time and headache by delving into the pros and cons of both.

Corporate World Pros:

1. Familiarity with Scope of Practice

In the corporate world, companies have more knowledge of what you can and cannot perform under your scope of practice. As a novel APRN, you may be asked to perform tasks that are not aligned with state licensure mandates, as each state has exceedingly specific delineations of duty, and larger corporations have invested their time and resources into ensuring these delineations are not being legally abused. The reason for this is mainly to decrease their potential for mitigation, which is definitely a pro for everyone.

2. Structured Orientation Programs

Doing business in a decent and orderly way is the chief aim of larger corporations. Again, the level of mastery a novel APRN is expected to have can be ensured when corporations invest in proper resources. As a novel APRN, it is usually refreshing to be reassured that one will not be "thrown to the wolves." Proper orientation gives the novel APRN sound validation on what is expected of him or her without ambiguity. This assurance is validating from both a competency and emotional standpoint.

3. Dedicated Supervision

In the corporate workplace, there is an illusion, if you will, that the corporation is invested in the success of the APRN (more on this to come later in the chapter) because there is usually assigned supervision for questions and collaboration. This can be a double-edged sword, but we will just focus on its positive aspects for now.

As a novel APRN, you enter the workforce with basic knowledge, and as a result, you may not recognize a hidden element of the subject matter, which can create a hazardous situation without guidance. I was once told by a nursing instructor early in my nursing training, "If you do not know what it is, you better know what it isn't." That little statement has stuck with me throughout my profession because, although it is a simple concept, it could not have been stated any better. Sometimes just knowing something is wrong can save you the headache of missing a potentially life-threatening diagnosis. Supervision helps identify those areas of clinical expertise that the novel APRN is not yet familiar with. Use that collaboration practice to your benefit as a novel APRN. It is greatly needed during this phase of your career.

4. Robust Legal Protection

The medical profession is one of the most litigious areas of practice among all occupations. Big corporations have full departments dedicated to protecting their assets. As an employee of a large corporation, you are considered an asset and, thus, are protected. That is *unless* you're practicing outside of the boundaries that have been set and structured by your workplace. In other words, *never cut corners*.

5. Peer Support

Peer support is just a fancy way of saying the novel provider will more than likely be working with multiple APRNs who can provide assistance. This extra layer of colleague support allows for brainstorming through medical or process (the method in which are done at a particular workplace) questions that one may not be as comfortable initially asking a physician counterpart. While this can be seen as a con, let us go ahead and count this as a pro coming from the novel APRN's perspective.

6. Guaranteed Pay Raise

Annual raises are wrapped in merit. Corporations are

very bureaucratic, which means processes flow in systematic order and are hardly ever personalized. One is usually always offered a nominal guaranteed rate increase followed by systematic benchmarks, allowing the more competitive or driven APRN to attain a higher increase. This is usually a good thing and can lead to job stability for the more enduring APRNs.

7. Incentive Packages (vacations, licensure, fees, CEU)

Corporations often package benefits nicely, which leads to competitiveness and attracts APRNs to the corporate world. One way of packaging benefits is by offering a salary and building on top of it with paid time off, vacations, sick time, and mandatory fee reimbursement (i.e., license, state pharmacy, federal DEA, liability, and CEU). Unfortunately, employers in the private sector usually cannot afford to guarantee these substantial benefits.

8. No Call or Guaranteed Fee for Call Services

The hospital does not close, so when a hospital employee's shift is over, preceding responsibilities are given to the relief until the person returns. Most corporate companies have dedicated call personnel, so employees can rest assured they will not be called at home with the progression of a patient's status after they've finished their workday. This is a strong pro that is not available in the private world.

The previously listed pros are all very appealing and sound great, but despite the attractiveness, there are some things that are not so easily identified in the corporate world. I like to refer to them as "traps."

Corporate World Cons:

1. Decreased Salaries

Usually because of the cost to maintain ancillary services, coupled with the offset in the cost of insurance and mandatory fees, employers will often offer the benefits packages previously listed. Yet, in all totality, you are paying for them out of your pocket. For example, instead of offering an employee a $100,000 salary, the employer will deduct the fees needed to fund your benefits package and offer you a salary of $85,000. Instead of getting a higher salary, the employee is offered a lower one with no capability to alter the incentive.

2. Workhorse Mentality

The corporate world usually mandates minimal workload quotas. For instance, it may be expected that the APRN sees thirty patients per day when working in a clinic, which puts them at risk of being reprimanded for not meeting their quota. Needless to say, this is in spite of the lack of control APRNs can be met with in the case of unforeseen circumstances.

3. The "All APRNs Are the Same and Come a Dime a Dozen" Mentality

There is little consideration for an individual's personal dilemmas. If workload quotas are not satisfied, there is a sense that you'll be replaced. If the APRN is not satisfied with their treatment in the workplace, which could be valid (i.e., mandatory overtime, inflexible schedule changes, etc.), one is made to feel that it's not a big deal to leave because a replacement can easily be located. This happens often in the corporate world, where the corporation touts what it has to offer and threatens to replace the employee if they fail to conform to the expectation, regardless of how realistic (or unrealistic) it may be.

4. Robust Condescending Physicians

Corporate physicians, especially when climbing up the proverbial ladder, are not ashamed of displaying their superiority. Often, the physician's demeanor may be condoned but not always appropriate, such as in a "good ol' boy system." There are exceptions to this in every workplace, but quite commonly, the physicians stick together. This is the number one reason APRNs are still bullied by physicians in the legislature, despite different governing boards.

5. Work Cattiness

Corporations with multiple employees oftentimes have cattiness that encompasses disgruntled "eat your own" nurses, physicians with superiority complexes (as mentioned above), work cliques, and gossip. This type of behavior is hardly ever entertained in a two-group practice, such as in a physician and NP relationship where there is a synergistic need for the other employee.

6. Decreased Acknowledgment of Degree Status

A nurse who, for instance, has climbed the chains from CNA to MA to LPN to RN to APRN, is immensely proud of their accomplishments. Despite how great this achievement is, some physicians, especially in the corporate world, still envision you as just a "nurse." There's a silent reminder that the physician's degree will always trump yours. So when decisions are being made regarding workflow, schedules, patient load, or personnel changes, it is often noted that the physician deems him or herself more valuable, diminishing your opinions by means of who is most valuable to the corporate world. Just think back to the many times you have heard that they will get rid of you, "the nurse," before the doctor.

7. Decreased Work Stability/Security

The notion of decreased work stability/security speaks for itself if you have understood the aforementioned sections. It is exceedingly difficult to feel a sense of work stability and security when one is made to feel devalued due to degree status or status quo.

8. Dedicated Supervision

Although this was previously listed as a pro, it can also be considered a con due to its dual action. To understand its negative implications, we must think of how the legislation has designed the collaborative practice for the APRN. It has been designed to always allow the physician a certain level of surveillance (notice I did not say oversight) over the APRN. While this may be necessary for a novel APRN, it is not required for an experienced APRN.

Because the CPA exists, some physicians believe it gives them the authority to dictate how APRNs document and treat a patient, even when the physician is incorrect. In the corporate world, especially hospitals, it is not uncommon for a physician to supervise an APRN's work and sometimes coerce or demand them to change things about their documentation or treatment plans. This is because they are overseeing the APRN. The physician can do this because most hospitals make it mandatory for the physician to sign all notes behind the APRN, regardless of the state law that requires only history, physical, and discharge summaries to be signed (pertaining to notes).

The APRN can stand firmly on personal documentation and observation yet still be made to change the note because the physician is not comfortable signing it as is. A situation such as this can create feelings of deflation or innate resentment in the APRN, which could potentially create an uncomfortable environment and further strain their job performance. It can be the start of a very tense working relationship if it's not appropriately addressed.

We have spent some time speaking about the corporate world, but it is now necessary to highlight the private world and what it offers. It seems corporate workplaces are popular for the reasons previously stated and their perceived stability, but there are quite a few pros that come with working in the private sector as well. It is only right that I identify them.

Private World Pros

1. *Personal One-on-One Training with a Physician*

When employed in the private world, one is usually employed by either a single physician or a small group of physicians. This intimacy provides a personal, typically one-on-one experience with a physician during the learning process. When paired with a credible, well-informed, and caring physician, the depth of knowledge shared is unimaginable.

2. *Autonomy*

This could easily be a pro if the NP is confident and understands there is always something to be learned. For the novel APRN, practicing autonomously can be challenging, but it *can* be achieved as long as the ARPN has the common sense to know when something does not add up. When this happens, the personal relationship between the physician and APRN blossoms into a positive and cooperative one, making it easy for the APRN to reach the physician for clarity and direction.

3. *Financial Advancement*

After years of limited work capabilities while maintaining clinical hours and classroom instruction (whether hybrid or in an actual classroom), a novel APRN can frequently be financially drained, with graduation, license, and testing fees added on top. In my personal experience, I was flat broke after I graduated. My first job was in the corporate sector, while some of my friends and colleagues decided to practice in the private world. Still, they were similarly financially broke. Now, it is to be noted that *some* of them faced financial hardships upon graduating, but certainly not all of them.

I can recall an incident where an NP working for a private physician needed a divorce and was able to get a loan from her boss to foot her problematic marriage that was affecting her work life. As novel APRNs, we do not enter these new roles looking for any assistance, but it is nice to have someone cover you if it's utterly necessary. This would *never* work (I know it is an absolute) in the corporate sector.

4. Having a Voice

As an APRN in the corporate world, decisions regarding your practice guidelines are generally made without your voice. There is usually a board comprised of your counterparts (APRNs or physician assistants) and administrative physicians who speak on your behalf. The problem with that is most providers in this role could not care less about your practice guidelines and have become very bureaucratic and cost-driven. Individuals in this role who make decisions on your behalf are compelled to think from more of a cost perspective and less from a patient-provider perspective.

Keeping this in mind, most APRNs do not have a voice in the corporate world; however, privately employed physicians usually care about your thoughts on how to improve the practice and what it will take to help you do your job better. Part of the logic for this is that a happy employee who has "bought in" to the practice model performs better. Performance is definitely a key factor for providers who rely on productivity to get reimbursed for services provided.

For instance, while on the clock at my first corporate job, the hospital medicine secretary, also known as the administrative assistant, quit. We were left without someone to distribute and assign patients by 6 a.m. Work, for me, started at 7 a.m. At the time, there were a total of six physicians and two NPs evenly split between rotations. The lead physician spoke with the other physicians and asked if anyone was interested in helping with this task; no one desired to do so. It was partially because a significant requirement of doing so meant awakening three to four hours before your shift started.

So, it was then decided that we, the APRNs, would be responsible. We did not have a choice. It became a pattern that whatever tasks the physicians did not desire to do, the APRNs had to do them, which made me feel devalued. I can only speak for myself, but when I feel devalued, I do not perform at my best because somehow, in my mind, I'm not a real team member; I'm more of the hired "dime a dozen" help. Needless to say, my honeymoon was over, my eyes were wide open, and I stayed for another three to four years before resigning. I had hoped to retire there.

Fast forward to my next job in the private sector. Before my first day of work, my new boss and I met up for dinner to discuss some expectations and my new role. He explained what time he started working and how his day flowed, then asked me what I thought my day would look like. I replied, "I think I would like to start my workday at 8 a.m." He replied, "That is more than reasonable." He also explained my choice of longer clinic hours Monday through Thursday with Friday off versus working shorter clinic hours Monday through Friday, with Fridays added to meet quotas.

I felt empowered to do well prior to even starting my first day because I interpreted his desire to take my decisions into consideration to mean I was valued and my decisions mattered. I am still employed with this physician, and he still asks for my input on practice-related concerns. While all private sector physicians are not like this, most value your input. This is commonly exhibited among my privately employed colleagues.

5. Increased Salaries

The private sector typically (not all-inclusive) supports a higher salary or 1099 employment where tax write-offs are more achievable. One can easily add $10,000 to $20,000 to their base salary in the private sector. This is an added value for APRNs with spouses who carry them on health insurance policies and do not need the health insurance benefit that is usually extremely attractive in the corporate world. Most APRNs who fit in this category prefer the bottom-dollar higher income that is not offered in the more rigid corporate world.

6. Less Work Cattiness

When working in the private sector, you often work alone or with one to two other APRNs, each of whom usually values the role and assistance of the other (provided each ARPN is responsible and communicative). The usual chatter, gossip, and increased potential for personality clashes that seem to accompany the corporate world are nearly completely diminished in smaller workplaces. This allows for less focus on emotionally draining aspects of the workplace and more productivity and learning, all of which improve you as a prudent APRN.

Hopefully, I have enlightened you regarding some of the pros of working in the private world. Despite this attractiveness, one must speak on those things that can be regarded as negative. In the private sector, the cons can feel a bit uneasy. Sometimes this is merely due to the lack of other employees to vent to (which can be a pro in itself). When experiencing a "negative" situation, one can feel alone. It is my goal to prepare you for some of the common uncomfortable situations in the private sector as an APRN. Remember, knowledge is half the battle.

Private World Cons

1. Longer Work Hours

When working for private physicians, you must be clear on the hours of operation, or rounding (also known as seeing patients). Often, these hours are not set in stone but, rather, are based upon the completion of duties. From the naked eye, this could appear to be a pro in the workforce, but physicians' reimbursements are dictated by how many people you see. So, naturally, the expectation of patients seen will be more than usual.

Private world physicians usually have the responsibility of clinic and hospital rounds. You may be expected to spend a set number of hours in the clinic while still being responsible for hospital rounds. Hospital rounds can encompass multiple facilities, all without accounting for travel time or gas. The autonomy of these roles seems appealing, but going day after day to satisfy the clinic hours (which cannot be altered), followed by travel time, gas, and spending time with each patient, can leave you working well over twelve hours daily. This does not seem like much when you factor in the fact that a nurse works twelve-hour days. But a nurse works three shifts per week, six per pay period, which is quite different from five or six twelve-hour shifts per week, ten to twelve per pay period.

So while the money seems great and the work, on the surface, is doable, it can be helpful to speak to APRNs who are already doing what you will be required to do and ask very strategic questions, like "Realistically, how many hours does it take you to complete your workday?" and "Do you have a lunch break?" In addition to those, asking, "How many times a week are you filling your car up to satisfy your requirements?" or even "Are you being compensated for gas or mileage?" are also really good questions.

When these questions are answered, consider whether you asked a seasoned APRN or a novel APRN. If your replies came from a seasoned APRN, double your time for several months until you become acclimated to your new role. I am sure after all is considered, you will agree with the decision to label work hours as a con.

2. Survival Practice

This section succinctly aligns with the previous one. If you can imagine working for yourself, payment is directly affected by the number of visits performed. Visits do not just apply to the home environment. Visits simply mean how many patients you have encountered in a single workday. This can be in the clinic, hospital, LTAC, skilled nursing facilities, or inpatient rehab units, to name a few. Private practices cannot financially survive without a workhorse mentality. The reason the APRN is responsible for rounds at multiple facilities is because employing an NP is only feasible if there are a number of facilities that need to be covered. The physician must gain something from hiring you (sad but true).

A common way APRNs help physicians is by covering more ground and seeing all of the patients prior to the physician's arrival. The APRN can aggregate the necessary patient information, such as lab results, vitals, and toleration/effects of medications, and write the note, thus drastically reducing the amount of time the physician needs to spend doing so. The physician can then stop by, review the data, speak briefly to the patient, and sign off on the notes, thereby creating more time for him or her to spend with family or see more patients.

Most physicians employ several NPs to cover more ground, increase their practice loads, and capitalize; however, some physicians will take on more responsibility and utilize the lone APRN by adding more to their workload. Be wary of this. This behavior is excellent if you are given a choice of added work and are compensated outside of the original agreement. If you are not, you can certainly end up abused and poorly compensated for your work due to time spent completing duties. When signing on or accepting employment from a single practicing physician, please be sure you get your contractual duties in writing. This gives you leverage to refuse additional assignments or calls without compensation.

I know I strayed off topic a little, but I just couldn't go without sharing that pearl of wisdom regarding contracts and how crucial they can be! Nevertheless, let's get back to the topic at hand.

Another survival practice con is that the privately practicing physician must see well over the usual corporate workload for the practice to survive and support multiple incomes. Be cautious when working with single practice physicians. Get everything in black and white (which hardly ever happens) before starting, and do not fall victim to what I call "survival work abuse."

3. Provider Pressure

In the last topic of survival practice, I mentioned that physicians will require more patient visits to support your salary. For the moment, the focus point will be the single practicing physicians who do not have partners but employ APRNs. For these physicians, survival is based solely on visits. Private employer physicians like the assistance of an APRN because they can double their workload and create more revenue; however, they can quickly forget, or are sometimes unaware of, the restraints the APRN may have in seeing some of the clientele the private physician may be capable of seeing. Keep in mind that the physician is not restricted from any practice duties, but the APRN is.

For example, my licensure state of Louisiana does not allow the APRN to prescribe medications for chronic pain or weight management, such as Adipex, or stimulants, such as Adderall, which are all highly sought after by patients and require monthly visits. There are a few exceptions to this with special board permission, but these are predominantly restricted functions of the APRN. For some physicians to financially survive, they will see chronic pain patients that cannot readily see a pain management physician due to insurance restrictions and limited availability of such specialty physicians. There is a vast population of people who genuinely require all phases of prescriptions for chronic pain, ADD/ADHD, or Adipex that falls in that insurance gap of limited specialty services available in their region. Some abusers fall under that same realm, and sometimes, the two are closely intertwined.

If those physicians are not careful, they can have a practice that's top-heavy with these sorts of patients. Because the physicians are trying to survive, they do not set a quota for such patient classes, especially when they have also employed an APRN. The physician then pressures the APRN to start seeing some of these patients because it increases visits, thereby increasing revenue.

Simply put, those physicians are trying to make ends meet. The problem is the APRN board prohibits such prescribing. If the physician is not careful, you can easily get pressured into seeing some of these chronic pain patients. A physician can say, "They have other co-morbid conditions you can treat; I will write for the pain medicine." This is completely legal, as the DEA allows such if the physician physically sees and examines the patient every fourth visit. Yet, suppose the wrong private physician employs you. In that case, you can end up seeing a patient without medical problems just for pain medications, despite the initial agreement that says you are not allowed to manage or prescribe. It is a gray area that can be uncomfortable, especially in the middle of an opioid crisis.

In a later chapter, I will outline steps for effective communication with the physician during uncomfortable situations.

4. No Guaranteed Raises

Unfortunately, it is fairly common for the APRN to work in the private world at their initial compensation rate for years without any mention of a pay raise. I would like to believe this is due to private employers' perceptions that it would be profligate to give pay raises when nothing about the financial dynamics of the workload or office has changed.

Let's say the hiring physician employs you as an APRN at $120,000 annually and you are made responsible for seeing forty patients per day. In a year or two, you would still be seeing an average of forty patients per day, and with no difference in the physician's bottom dollar to incentivize him or her to pay you more, your wage has been capped at that initial $120,000 annual rate.

Naturally, I would suggest combating this. If you found yourself employed by a private physician or group, discuss annual raises in the hiring contract and get the specifics written in black and white.

5. Health Care, Vacation, and Insurance Costs

Frequently, when hired by a private physician or group, salaries are slightly higher, but they usually do not include health insurance, life insurance, 401K investment capabilities, or liability insurance costs. For those persons covered under their spouse's packages, this is likely not a big deal for you, except for liability insurance, which is a big deal for all practicing APRNs. Sometimes the physician will umbrella you under his or her liability insurance, but you will have to be sure about this before starting.

Speaking of liability insurance, if you must obtain your own policy, make sure you converse with other APRNs first so you do not cheat yourself in the process. Liability insurance is not like car insurance in that you can search for the most competitive rates, which is particularly important to protect yourself. God forbid you get sued, but the probability is high, regardless of your skill level. We live in a very litigious world where many people are looking for ways to receive a monetary advancement rather expeditiously or, as I like to say, are looking for a quick "come up."

When searching for liability insurance, pay attention to the reviews. Seek recommendations from your nurse practitioner association and colleagues who have been involved in litigation. Always, always, always get what is called a "tail" policy. I'm stressing its importance because liability insurance without a tail component does not cover you for any cases that occurred while you were employed once you leave a job. This means if you work for a physician or company for ten years and quit tomorrow, you will not be covered for any lawsuits that arise even if the incident occurred while you were still employed.

Let me clarify this with an example. Suppose I take care of "patient X" on December 15, 2019, while employed at Mercy Hospital, which was covered under my policy. In June of 2020, I quit Mercy Hospital and, a month later, get notification of a lawsuit involving "patient X". Without tail coverage, I am no longer covered by that previous insurance policy, though I was covered when the incident occurred back in December 2019.

Most of us know lawsuits are lengthy, and sometimes intent to sue notifications happen months or years later. Without tail coverage, you are essentially, for lack of a better term, screwed. This is something I think should be taught more in the actual APRN program.

While that information was just too important to not caveat, we must get back on topic. Make sure you ask important questions during the hiring phases, especially regarding liability coverage. Though most of these incentive packages are not available in the private employment sector, sometimes they exist.

6. Autonomy Abuse

This is an important topic. I am sure you are thinking, *What is autonomy abuse?* This is when a private physician has an extraordinarily strong APRN delegated to do rounds at various LTAC, SNF, and IPR hospitals. Technically, according to the regulations of the hospital bylaws and for the sake of scope of practice for the APRN, in these acute care hospitals and LTAC facilities, the physician should be rounding behind the APRN. Sometimes, however, the physician will get too comfortable with the level of trust garnered for the APRN. The physician trusts the APRN's judgment, becomes complacent, and never shows up to round behind them. This leaves the APRN vulnerable and practicing outside of the scope against their will.

Regardless of the comfort level, the APRN should mostly be concerned with the precarious position this puts them in from a licensing and governing board perspective. APRNs in the state of Louisiana (check your state's governing practice guidelines) cannot practice independently; however, they can own a clinic and practice in collaboration with a physician. In this instance, the physician does not have to be on-site but merely audit a limited amount of records per month.

However, in the hospital and LTAC world, the physician is mandated to be more "present."

Acute care environments, like the hospital, require daily physician presence, but in the LTAC world, rounds can be done daily by the APRN and at least a couple times a week by the physician. Some physicians will round daily in the LTAC for reimbursement purposes (this will be explained later), but the physician can likely get away with not seeing the patient every day (someone must see the patient daily out of you two), as long as it is not billed as if they have. Still, the physician certainly must show up at least a couple of times a week in addition to collaborating with the APRN who may be seeing the patient daily.

What I am trying to convey is some physicians will get comfortable with the clinically strong APRN and never show up, leaving the APRN self-practicing, which should never happen. At this point, the physician is abusing the work autonomy of the APRN, which causes them to become vulnerable from a litigious and governing standpoint. This is a sticky situation because the APRN's license may be compromised, and quitting the job may be the only feasible solution to avoid such a thing from happening if they cannot get the physician to show up.

If you are in a position like this but have not decided how to handle the situation, please confirm that the physician is not billing for services as if they have seen the patient. The reimbursements are different and can unknowingly place you in a fraudulent situation. If the physician does not see the patient, the patient *must* be billed under an APRN visit (which is 85 percent reimbursement) rather than a physician visit (which is 100 percent reimbursement). You do not want to get in a situation with the FBI where they are showing up and interviewing you for fraudulent billing. It is an uncomfortable situation to be in, regardless of your knowledge on the matter. Sometimes ignorance is not enough.

Knowledge is power. Be informed. Ask tough questions. And speak with your physician about how autonomy abuse is affecting you. If the behavior is not changed, quit to protect your license and your sanity. The monetary gain is not worth the headache if you get audited by the board or the federal government.

In closing this chapter, I do not think there is a right or wrong answer to which setting, whether corporate or private, you choose. Every individual is different and has needs that are unique to them. If you are married and carried under your spouse's insurance, deciding to go with a higher-paying job that does not offer health insurance but offers tail end liability insurance seems reasonable. If you are a novel APRN who wants more structure and educational support, the corporate world would probably be more suitable. Whatever decision you make, remember to be well informed and ask tough questions during the interview phase as outlined in this chapter. The answers will ultimately help you with whatever you are trying to accomplish in the long run.

Recap: Here is a chart of pros and cons per the career settings previously discussed:

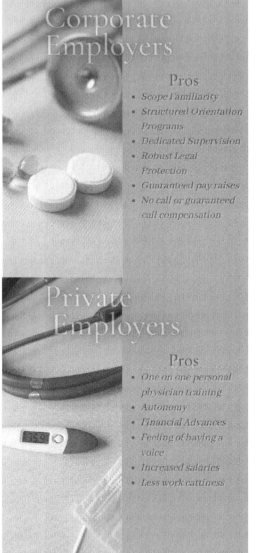

Corporate Employers

Pros

- Scope Familiarity
- Structured Orientation Programs
- Dedicated Supervision
- Robust Legal Protection
- Guaranteed pay raises
- No call or guaranteed call compensation

Cons

- Decreased salaries
- Workhorse mentality
- Dime a dozen mentality
- Condescending physicians
- Work cattiness
- Decreased acknowledgement of degree status
- Decreased feeling of job security

Private Employers

Pros

- One on one personal physician training
- Autonomy
- Financial Advances
- Feeling of having a voice
- Increased salaries
- Less work cattiness

Cons

- Longer work hours
- Survival practice behavior
- Provider pressure
- No guaranteed raises
- Healthcare, Vacation, and Liability insurance costs
- Autonomy abuse

3
KNOW YOUR SCOPE OF PRACTICE

In APRN school, there is a semester dedicated to healthcare policy. This is when the scope of practice is usually discussed. In my personal opinion and experience, NP students do not fully understand most of what is highlighted during this particular phase of the program. Because of this, NPs are not fully aware of what they can and cannot do upon graduation and job attainment. There is so much excitement in school completion, graduation, and attaining their first role as an NP that one can forget about the scope until they're actually on the job in their new role as a healthcare provider. There will be major red flags and common-sense actions that a novel APRN will know better than to do, like prescribe to friends or family members, but the novel APRN will soon realize there are a lot of gray areas. What is even more mind-blowing is that some (not all) fellow nurses will attempt to downgrade your success by pointing out the things you cannot do.

Before my first job, I was not made aware of what I call "professional jealousy." I can vividly recall my initial experience with this type of behavior. It was very jarring and occurred on my very first job as an emergency room APRN, which was surprisingly very antiquated for the NP. I suspect there was a board of physicians who wrote the policies of what the emergency medicine APRN could and could not perform at that hospital. Although the state requires physician collaboration and I had an agreement signed by multiple ED physicians, that hospital did not allow me, as an emergency room NP, to collaborate with the physician; instead, I reported to the ED nurse manager. I was limited to empiric medical treatment only, which meant that upon assessment of a patient, I could not order any diagnostic testing other than a urinalysis (I am not making this up). So if a patient came in with abdominal pain and I believed they required workup, such as CT imaging, plain film imaging, or ultrasounds, I had to ask the RN in charge to speak with the ER physician or ask the ER charge nurse to reroute that patient to the physician. This is an example of purposefully limiting the APRN.

Allow me to provide another example. One day, at the same hospital mentioned above, I was lucky enough to run into one of the ED doctors. I expressed feeling limited and wanting to, at the very least, be able to hone in on my I&D skills. I asked the physician if I could come to his side and perform I&Ds when I wasn't busy. He excitedly stated, "Yes, I'll let you know when we get some." The charge RN was listening, and later that day, when speaking to another RN who had been working in that particular ED for over ten years, she talked about me as if I was not present. She basically let the other RN know that the physician said I could do I&Ds, but she didn't believe that was in my scope, so she saw to it that I would not be able to do them. I quit that job the next day. This is an instance of potential professional jealousy from your nursing counterparts.

Again, some nurses (not all) will be upset that you actually went back to school and finished. "How dare you?" is the kind of connotation that can be present in some environments. Beware and try not to feed into the drama. Pick your battles and know that if pettiness is a part of the general environment of the facility, you probably won't be able to change the behavior alone. However, you can prove to them you are above it by ignoring it and letting your work speak for itself. If it had not been for the limited scope of practice at that facility, I would have stayed, but the liability of empiric treatment in an acute care environment that had access to comprehensive testing for rule-outs was too much for me to tolerate, along with the nursing culture.

That behavior was not present at all in the job following that encounter, so please do not get me wrong. All nurses are not professionally jealous of the APRN. Some confident nurses are genuinely proud of you, but there are many who "eat their young" daily. Beware of the nurses who will try to make you feel like you are incapable of assessing, diagnosing, and prescribing.

Some physicians may also remind you of what you cannot do, but *only* when it is for their benefit. If you, as the APRN, do not take anything else away from this chapter, take away the fact that *most* physicians are clueless about your limitations as an APRN. Each state has an advanced practice governing board under the umbrella of the registered nursing board in your country. Your scope can be found in your nurse practice act. Please refer to your state's scope of practice for guidance. If nothing else, inform yourself and try not to allow anyone to educate you on what your scope is. If

I had a dollar for every duty I've been asked to do outside of my scope, I would be rich. When I reply to a physician, "I would love to be a team player and help you with the certain duty or action requested, but cannot because of my board-outlined scope," the reply is usually, "Why not? Why can't you do it?" or "I didn't know that." This is especially common among private physicians who hire APRNs. Common out-of-scope requests include broadening your patient clinic census to include Adderall/Adipex patients, seeing chronic pain patients, and signing physician-only attestation forms for the MD because the physician did not have time to stop at the facility that needs the papers signed.

It is OK to be flexible in other ways. Work with your collaborators to get things done, but *never* compromise your license in the process. I have offered to get the paperwork, take it to the physician, and bring it back. You do not have to go out of your way to help with this, but the flexibility will take you a long way. Get to know your physician if you are working in the private sector and decide if they are worthy of your flexibility. If the answer is no, then find a new job because that place of employment will most likely be miserable if you cannot form a bond with the person you will work closest with. The relationship will determine your flexibility and enhance your growth. The MDs offer so much for novel APRNs to learn from.

Something nifty about Louisiana, the state where I practice, is that if you are confused about any action request, you can call the board and speak with an APRN representative who will help guide you. Remember, it is very typical for most of your hiring agents or leadership to not be aware of your scope of practice *unless* you are being employed with a major magnet status or equivalent corporation.

4
CHASING THE DOLLAR

It is fantastic to come out of school, usually broke, and get your hustle on, but be wary of what I call "chasing the dollar." Most companies with large scales of pay have many more demands and heavier workloads. This is not a bad thing, but be clear of what you will and will not do for that dollar.

Imagine a hypothetical scenario where a new graduate is offered $130,000 annually but is required to see twenty patients per day in clinic (which is very difficult to manage for a novel APRN who's still learning a new role, new workplace, and new coworkers). In addition to this, the graduate has to drive to three hospitals that are twenty to twenty-five minutes away from each other to see hospitalized patients. It is often true that the demands usually support the income.

Some gems will not require such enormous demands, so I am not saying an excellent salary as a new grad is not possible. I am saying to know what the expectation is before signing up *just* for the dollar. It will save you a lot of headaches, burnout, and disgruntled emotions.

It is essential to know what your expectations are. Can you imagine making great money but being unhappy and feeling like you have to stay because you cannot afford to leave? This is a common pitfall of chasing the dollar. Chase what you love as it pertains to being an APRN, and yes, you will have bad days, but they will never be regretful days. When we stay at a job we hate because the money is good, we have, in all essence, become a slave to the dollar. Also, when we have become accustomed to working multiple APRN jobs to regularly support the material things we want (and then cannot quit working some of those jobs due to overhead that demands you stay), you have become a slave to the dollar.

Let me give an illustration. You work two jobs to save for the down payment on your dream house. You then buy the house but keep the second job to furnish it. You buy the furniture, then keep the job for a new car. You get the new car and continue to work over one hundred hours a week because you do not know how to give up the extra income *or* you have incurred significant debt (inflated mortgage, hefty car notes, substantial credit card debt) that requires you keep it. So you now have worked one-hundred-plus hours per week for over five years, and there is no clear end to it, but you are burned out. You are officially a slave to the dollar!

This is extremely easy to become trapped in. Be clear about the work-life balance you want. Be calculated with working extra for a goal. Make it meaningful to you. If you're going to hustle and are comfortable with always working two jobs, this chapter is not for you. It is for the NP who can potentially let debt due to lifestyle creep up and control them and now *must* work two or more jobs to survive. APRN responsibilities are mostly mental and not very physical. It is excellent that you are no longer "killing your back," but trust, that mental work is much more taxing. You do not want to mentally exhaust yourself.

I will repeat: be calculating and purposeful with your career choices and work-life balance. If you are someone who is not good at managing money, invest in a financial planner or a competent certified public accountant, preferably a distinguished one. I see this particular issue so often in many of my colleagues and, truthfully, a little in myself. With that being said, be informed, be calculated, and be purposeful in protecting your financial, mental, and physical health.

5
HOW TO MARKET YOURSELF

I briefly spoke on the interview-to-employment process in chapter one. It is not a quick process. The typical time frame between employment and the first day of work is three to six months in the corporate world and one to two months in the private world, so start looking for your new job during your last semester. This may seem a little audacious because you must still graduate and pass boards, but if you made it to the last semester, you know what it takes to graduate and pass. You are resilient, so have faith in yourself and start looking. Trust me on this; you'll thank me later.

Only apply for positions you can realistically see yourself doing. Do your homework and speak to other NPs about prospective places of employment (only if you trust them), but form your own opinion. This means do not allow another peer's opinion to become yours. Your questions to peers about the reputation of a potential employer should only be used to guide your questions for the interview process. If you do not get anything else out of this chapter, get that you should not apply to anyplace you *do not* want to work. If you shoot for peanuts, you'll get peanuts, so be clear about what you want.

Join the local nurse practitioner association in your area and network; get to know people. It is easiest to find out which establishments are looking to add to their roster from individuals who are already employed at the potential hiring location. These individuals (i.e., actively working ARPNs) are usually members of their local nurse practitioner organization, so use these organizations to your advantage. Additionally, it is much cheaper to join as a student.

Know what the going market rate is for the APRN. It varies from state to state and city to city and follows the same rules as supply and demand. If the market is saturated, the salary will be lower. This is mainly because most corporations employ the notion that APRNs come "a dime a dozen." A realistic average for a novel APRN's base salary in Louisiana is roughly $90,000 to $100,000 annually in the corporate world and $100,000 to $120,000 annually in the private world. Keep potential demands in mind and be prepared to be precise and calculated in your questions. The base salary for the corporate sector usually does not include bonuses.

If a physician in the private world asks whether you want to be paid per patient or a fixed salary, consider that if you take a per-patient-based pay as a full-time employee, your checks will significantly decrease during slower times. Patient-based pay is something to consider for supplemental income but should be avoided for full-timers unless you have done your homework and know for a fact that your physician has a consistent amount of patients. It is important to mention that even hospitals slow down, so proceed with caution for full-time employers.

If you consider per-patient employment, the going rate should be higher in hospitals. Physicians are paid based on patient accrual. Do not settle. Market yourself for hospital versus NH rates. NH reimbursements are considerably lower than the hospital. This is an estimation, but based upon some unofficial inquiries to friends on the billing and collection side in Louisiana, the physician, regardless of billing, will get an average of $50 per progress note on each acute care patient seen and documented. The physician will also get $25 per nursing home patient (give or take). The term acute care encompasses hospital, LTAC, and inpatient rehab. Skilled and nursing homes go hand in hand from a billing standpoint. Remember, these rates are prior to biller fees and overhead, so when considering your fee for patients seen (if you choose that route), you can loosely use these fees as a guide.

I have included a table at the end of this chapter that outlines the APRN's average salary per state (from low to high) based on this book's initial publication date. Please keep in mind that multiple factors influence salary ranges, and thus, this table is not all-inclusive. Some factors to consider include certification type and other qualifications, such as CCRN certification, the ability to speak different languages, et cetera.

Be confident when selling yourself and marketing what you have to offer. Your knowledge and background experience will determine how valuable you are to the physician or company. Speak objectively and always look your potential employers in the eye. If you get a bad vibe, trust your gut; it is called discernment.

SALARY COMPARISON CHART

Practice State	Salary Range (from low to high)	Median Salary (per state)
Alabama	$82,254 – $101,733	$90,034
Alaska	$98,406 – $121,711	$107,714
Arizona	$86,790 – $107,343	$94,999
Arkansas	$80,960 – $100,133	$88,618
California	$98,055 – $121,276	$107,330
Colorado	$87,521 – $108,247	$95,800
Connecticut	$94,983 – $117,476	$103,967
District of Columbia	$97,642 – $120,766	$106,879
Delaware	$92,173 – $114,002	$100,892
Florida	$83,395 – $103,145	$91,283
Georgia	$84,931 – $105,045	$92,965
Hawaii	$92,103 – $113,915	$100,815
Idaho	$82,853 – $102,474	$90,690
Illinois	$90,154 – $111,505	$98,682
Indiana	$85,765 – $106,076	$93,878
Iowa	$84,010 – $103,905	$91,956
Kansas	$83,307 – $103,036	$91,187
Kentucky	$82,605 – $102,167	$90,419

Louisiana	$84,097 – $104,013	$92,052
Maine	$84,624 – $104,665	$92,629
Maryland	$90,511 – $111,945	$99,072
Massachusetts	$95,509 – $118,128	$104,544
Michigan	$87,854 – $108,660	$96,165
Minnesota	$89,803 – $111,070	$98,298
Mississippi	$76,372 – $94,459	$83,596
Missouri	$83,658 – $103,470	$91,572
Montana	$79,746 – $103,579	$87,104
Nebraska	$80,498 – $99,562	$88,113
New Hampshire	$89,101 – $110,202	$97,529
New Jersey	$97,054 – $120,038	$106,235
New Mexico	$80,235 – $99,236	$87,824
Nevada	$89,979 – $111,288	$98,490
New York	$94,192 – $116,499	$103,102
North Carolina	$83,746 – $103,579	$91,668
North Dakota	$82,429 – $101,950	$90,226
Ohio	$85,713 – $106,011	$93,820
Oklahoma	$82,517 – $102,059	$90,323
Oregon	$87,433 – $108,139	$95,703
Pennsylvania	$87,609 – $108,356	$95,896
Rhode Island	$92,525 – $114,436	$101,277
South Carolina	$82,166 – $101,625	$89,938
South Dakota	$75,143 – $92,939	$82,251

Tennessee	$79,752 – $98,639	$87,296
Texas	$86,201 – $106,616	$94,355
Utah	$83,169 – $102,865	$91,037
Vermont	$84,536 – $104,556	$92,533
Virginia	$87,258 – $107,922	$95,511
Washington	$93,754 – $115,956	$102,622
West Virginia	$77,777 – $96,196	$85,134
Wisconsin	$86,467 – $106,945	$94,647
Wyoming	$78,121 – $96,630	$85,518

Information in chart provided by "Advanced Practice Nurse Salary" Salary.com, www.salary.com/research/salary/recruiting/advanced-practice-nurse-salary. Accessed 8 Aug. 2020.

6
STAY IN YOUR LANE

It is essential to know your strengths and limitations. Most APRN students choose a family focus to be marketable and not confined to one role. But being marketable starts long before your choice of concentration. Many factors, including market saturation, determine your appeal to the employer and in the overall market.

For instance, if there are two APRN openings but one thousand applicants, what do you think is being utilized to determine who gets an interview? If you guessed background, you've hit the nail on the head. Your background should match your concentration focus. For instance, a mother-baby RN is more likely to land a secure job as a neonatal or pediatric-based NP over family, despite the ability of the family trained APRN to provide care to the neonate. This does not mean a long-standing mother-baby RN should not decide to try something outside of their element; rather, they should strengthen their resume *before* graduating as an FNP.

My advice would be to work in a medical-surgical unit

at a well-respected hospital one or two days a week while gaining your FNP. Have something to offer the employer that makes them confident in their ability to train you as a novel APRN. Go above and beyond to show you are dedicated to your new role. If you do not desire to swap positions in the middle of ARPN school, try asking your hospital if you can shadow an FNP in the ICU at your hospital outside of your clinical rotation. This alternative is problematic for most NP students because, realistically, how does one find additional time to volunteer outside of work demands and mandatory clinical rotation? This is why a role conversion prior to graduation is more realistic.

Do what you must do to show your potential new employer that you deserve that job over the other FNP candidates. And if you do not want to do the work to remain marketable, stay in your lane or use networking to get in the door in a new and unfamiliar area of expertise.

7

INTERVIEW COMMUNICATION

When interviewing, as previously stated, do your homework and be clear about your expectations. Interviews are a two-way conversation. Please be professional and courteous. It is OK to jot down key points and questions to ask later so the interviewer can finish their thought. The more you are informed about the company or physician beforehand, the more ahead of the game you are. Do your homework. Before you approach the interview, know what the mean salary is for the position you are applying for.

Does this employer meet your expectations? What are the expectations of you as a novel APRN? What are some perks and incentives for gaining your employment? How long is the training for a novel APRN, and to whom do you report? Once you get the answer to all your questions, take some time to reflect on what you are asking for and whether or not it aligns with your requesting salary. In other words, are your expectations realistic? Go back to the median salary chart at the end of chapter five if you're not sure. If you're not realistic, you will likely remain on the hamster wheel of interviewing without gaining employment. Do not cheat yourself out of an excellent salary, but more importantly, do not cheat yourself out of a great opportunity; the money will come. As a novel APRN, always choose the experience over the money. Trust me on this one.

8

Does the Work Match the Pay? (Know Your Worth While Knowing Your Limitations)

It will be an immensely proud moment when you land that marvelous job that pays handsomely. I applaud you in advance for putting in the work to get that high-paying job. Enjoy your honeymoon, and be cautious of the silent, unforeseen duties that may arise. Be careful about accepting additional duties without compensation, as you can easily get overwhelmed, grow to hate your role, and become annoyed with your employer.

In my own experience, I had a job that was marketed as having a great work-life balance. It promised more time with my family, as the employer knew I was working ten-hour days at my previous job. The job quickly went from eight hours daily for fourteen consecutive days before getting an off day to over twelve hours daily with increased workloads and calls. In addition to this, I was still working fourteen days consecutively. Now, mind you, my previous job was ten-hour days seven on and seven off. This meant I never worked more than fourteen days per month. This new job easily quadrupled my workload.

Although it sounds like a setup, I was compensated for every additional duty, so this job turned out to be a financial dream despite the hefty workload. However, not everyone wants to work like a workhorse, and those people should be mindful of what they are getting into before one day awakening to realize they do not have a life. This is especially important because if the realization that you may have bitten off more than you can chew sets in, you may be stuck in that position due to the fear of financial instability.

Realistically, if it sounds too good to be true, it probably is. Talk to other colleagues, be informed, and ask difficult questions, which brings us to the next chapter: how to effectively communicate during a difficult situation.

9

EFFECTIVE COMMUNICATION WITH YOUR PHYSICIAN OR EMPLOYER WHEN YOU ARE UNCOMFORTABLE

It is amazingly simple to communicate when one is comfortable with the topic or when the conversation is favorable, but there will be instances when it's imperative to speak up for yourself, though you should do so without giving off a tone of aggression or pessimism. Over the years of professional nursing in multiple management roles and then as a novel to now seasoned APRN, it has become evident that when speaking up, the message is often overlooked by the delivery. It is imperative to remain even-toned and mind your feelings when conversing or discussing uncomfortable situations.

Regardless of how emotional the topic becomes or how the conversation makes you feel, maintaining composure and thinking about what you want to relay to your audience most should be the highest priority. This composure can be the single factor that determines the outcome of what you are trying to convey and how it is perceived. When presented with this scenario, we, as passionate advocates, must check our feelings at the table of the conversation until there is time to think and organize our thoughts accordingly. Your tone and delivery should match your degree of professionalism. I will list some instances when speaking up is imperative, but overall, delivery is monumental and crucial for positive outcomes.

Scenario One:

The physician asks you to perform a task that is outside of your scope, illegal, or unsafe. When one works for a physician who exudes intimidation or when the APRN is fearful of being terminated, it is difficult to effectively articulate to a physician that there is uneasiness in performing a particular requested duty.

Let's say you are managing a hospitalized observation patient who has chest pain and a history of ESRD on HD. The patient has elevated cardiac markers, which may be baseline considering his ESRD. This hospital presentation shows baseline markers but is presenting chest pain differently. The physician performs a quick overview of the patient data and tells you to discharge them. Although you are a novel APRN, you have performed the history of presenting illness and physical exam and believe this presentation is different from usual and may indicate a true cardiac issue. You are uncomfortable discharging the patient but are not sure how to address it.

Scenario Two:

You are working in a private physician-owned clinic where numbers drive the business. The geographic location has resulted in physicians performing low-level chronic pain management. Low-level means the number of narcotics is written at a level under the radar of what is considered alarming. However, patients return monthly for refills. This task is usually performed at a chronic pain site, not primary care. The physician is doing this in an attempt to survive, seeing more than what is comfortable for a primary care facility.

You, as a novel APRN, are seeing primary care patients without the need for chronic pain management, mainly because the licensing board has restricted chronic pain management from the APRN (thank God!). However, while your boss, collaborator, or physician is the one who will be writing the pain scripts, you may be requested to see some of these patients. You are uncomfortable with performing this duty but are unsure how to articulate it.

Scenario Three:

A clinically strong APRN works in the private sector and rounds at multiple facilities for a single physician. The physician's sole responsibility is to show up to the facility several times a week at minimum. The physician recognizes the APRN's strengths and feels comfortable enough to not show up at the facilities, thus the APRN is left unintentionally practicing outside of their scope.

This particular situation once happened to a friend of mine, and it occurs in the private world often. It is easily an unintentional vehicle to practice beyond your scope. It is clearly a gray area because the APRN has no other option than to quit if the physician's duties are not performed. Without cooperation from the physician, the APRN is vulnerable.

In all three scenarios, articulation in a non-confrontational and even tone, along with objectively taking one's feelings out of the conversation, is optimal and, in most cases, highly effective. One must state the harm the behavior is causing or how it affects one's licensure.

The best way to communicate is face-to-face with concrete, verifiable data, like, say, an article that reflects what one's scope is. This way of communication is useful for private-sector employees. For corporate world employees, it is the same presentation combined with the addition of a polite request for a meeting in writing so a paper trail is created. *Always* have documented evidence of what the conversation is about so there is no room for the corporate world big wigs, as I like to call them, to work against you. You must not speak to anyone else about your issues in the corporate or private world. Speak directly with the physician or corporate supervisor. Making more individuals aware of the situation will only complicate matters and create unintentionally heightened awareness. Be careful not to become the sounding board for those who may have similar experiences but are too afraid to speak up. Remember to speak on what negatively affects *you*, not everyone else. Pick your battles.

These examples are matters that can affect licensure and must involve a non-provoking, calm conversation where self-control and factual data is the only thing being presented. Speak objectively, and it should go well. If it affects your license and the physician (private world) or chains of command (corporate world) are not listening, your workplace is now hostile. Protect your license and professionally resign. Often, factual data without the exhibition of passion is impactful and creates change *and* respect.

10
SAFE PRACTICE

This chapter briefly explains dos and don'ts for the novel APRN. I will only speak briefly about this topic, as there will be further published guides on safe practice. This is merely information on how to guide your practice as a novel APRN. Here are a few pointers:

Do develop trust with your patients.

The patient's level of trust will determine what is divulged to you as a practitioner. Oftentimes, patients hold back information that is integral in treating them because they do not want to feel judged or they are unsure of your authenticity. Despite making an appointment with you as a provider, this is an interview process for them, so be aware that the patient is also interviewing you. They are observing your demeanor, genuineness, and display of interest in their issues. In addition to this, they are also taking note of your exhibition of empathy toward their problems. If you can follow a few simple steps, you will build a rapport with your patient, which will go a long way with getting the necessary information to treat them.

Be nonjudgmental and maintain eye contact with engaging behavior. Look at your patient when you speak to them, as it exudes respect and interest. Avoid typing notes while listening to them. Sit (the closer to them, the better) rather than stand over them. Do not cut them off, regardless of whether the conversation appears to be delusional or fictitious. Avoid redirection in the initial visit. Clarify what you may not understand.

Don't talk condescendingly to your patient, even if it is frustrating to interact with them.

Sometimes patients will want to speak a lot or they may have issues they feel are paramount and want to discuss them in detail. Listen to them, even if, as a provider, you may know or believe their problems are insignificant or downright fictitious. There are two things to keep in mind: 1) Patients are sometimes elusive, and 2) at the time of this guide's publication, we are in the middle of an opioid crisis. Despite your initial feelings on your conversation with the patient, avoid talking over them or being dismissive or condescending.

Frequently, as the provider, we must reiterate what a patient states and back up the non-logical portion of their conversation with data without saying flat-out that the patient's problem is, in fact, nonfactual or unbelievable. Avoid attempts to convince a patient that their information is fictitious unless you have formed a solid rapport with them. Otherwise, you will not convince them, so save your breath.

As a society, we are all different. Diversity and individual differences are what make the world rotate. Enjoy those varieties and try to understand the misfortunate, the drug addict, the manipulator, and the poor. Not all patients will be "good," clean-cut, or upstanding citizens with excellent backgrounds. They still matter. Instead of writing them off completely, be objectively stern with the drug addict. Have nonnegotiables in your practice or utilize the office or workplace policies that prevent you from getting stuck writing a bunch of narcotics scripts. You still must be receptive to a valid medical necessity, so know the difference. And if the patient's clinical exam does not indicate the need for what they've requested, remain calm and avoid being condescending. You may be the difference in what makes a patient move on with the day, overcome depression, or commit suicide. Always display a caring demeanor and avoid judging patients; this will go a long way.

Try to ascertain why your patient may not be adherent. Dig deep. As a dedicated medical provider, avoid expressing your frustration at the patient's perceived unwillingness to do what you desire, even if it benefits them. I cannot stress this enough: *Dig deep*. Don't be afraid to be direct. Go ahead and ask, "Why are you not taking your medication or failing to check your blood pressure or capillary glucose levels?"

It is true you will have patients who are downright and blatantly non-adherent. But there is a large amount of patients who want to do the right thing but have barriers in doing so. It is an understatement to simply say, "Pay attention to your patient." Often, we have an ancillary staff to obtain vital signs, confirm the medication list, and obtain chief complaints. Please go over this with your patient. You are the *trained* provider who will pick up on things the patient may not feel comfortable admitting to the ancillary staff or even you.

One time, I had a patient with persistently uncontrolled HTN. I saw the patient weekly for BP checks and medication evaluations to get their blood pressure controlled. Every visit, my medical assistant would go over his home meds for changes or omissions. He never had any. Despite the increase in dosage and the addition of BP meds, his blood pressure remained elevated. Finally, I asked the patient how many pills he was taking, and he replied, "Everything you give me." That response was too broad.

As a provider, I did not get frustrated. I simply asked him to pull out his medication. Although he stumbled a bit, he retrieved the bottle of pills from his pocket and handed it to me. I then held the bottle up and asked him if he was taking it once or twice a day. He struggled to provide an answer, despite having the frequency of dosage typed on the bottle by the pharmacist. It had finally dawned on me that he could not read. Though that was an initial question asked during the interview process, the patient did not feel comfortable initially divulging that information, so he did not. After forming a rapport with the patient, I asked, "Can you read?" He jokingly replied, "You know people from the country can't read."

After this discovery, I was able to work with him and color-coded his daytime medication bottles blue and his nighttime bottles black. He understood this and complied with treatment. The following week, his blood pressure was controlled. Initially, I was quite perturbed with my MA for not tuning into the fact that the patient could not read until I realized the anger I had for my MA was misplaced. I was actually annoyed with myself. Some things are better left undelegated. The lesson I learned was to collect sensitive information myself instead of delegating it to my staff, regardless of what the clinic or corporate policy was.

Patients can be non-adherent to meds and treatment for multiple reasons, including financial constraints, pure ignorance, fear, self-neglect due to sick parents or special needs kids, depression, or a lack of confidence in the provider. Show your patients you care, and they will divulge.

There is a flip side to this to avoid being a sounding board during each visit, but that will be discussed in another volume. First, as a novel provider, you must learn to tune your ear and have a keen eye for assessment. Developing these skills will take you further in your career than learning when to redirect the interview or visit. Time will teach you those skills for the most part.

Never form an opinion about a patient based on what another provider says, even if you're friends with them or related to them. Instead, it is always best to *talk* with your patient and form your own opinion. I would be remiss if I didn't acknowledge the fact that every patient will not be tolerable, so pick your battles. If you have a patient you just cannot think positively about, ask to switch them to another provider or fire them. Save yourself a headache and a lawsuit. Suppose you missed or failed to treat something in a patient because your annoyance with them made it rather difficult to listen to them effectively. In that case, *you* will regret it both emotionally and financially. The same applies to patients. When they do not feel heard, they move on to new providers.

The first questions I ask patients to establish care are "Who was your last provider?" and "Why did you leave?" Often, the patients will have practical reasons as to why they decided to seek another provider. Asking questions like this is an excellent way to feel the patient out while you are being reviewed as well.

Remember when I spoke of patients who may be hard to listen to due to perceived fictional components of their story (though you should still hear them out)? This is the stage where you will figure out if your patient is reasonable or not. This is the optimum time for both sides to map out their expectations. Keep in mind that establishment of care appointments are a two-way interview and are essential in building a successful practice.

Do listen to your patient but avoid generalizations.

When speaking with your patient during the interview phase of HPI, avoid generalizations on both your end and the patient's end. For instance, if your patient has diabetes mellitus, you inquire how their glucose levels are, and the patient responds with something like, "They've been good." Ask them exactly what "good" quantifies. The provider's definition of "good" is more than likely different from the patient's. If the patient is accustomed to glucose levels of 400 mg/dl, "good" to them may be a level of 300 mg/dl. If you do not hone in on exact measurements, there could be a lack of treatment you, as a provider, will be held liable for. The same stands true for blood pressures, alcohol or tobacco abuse, and so much more. Make sure your patient provides information in a quantifiable manner.

Another valuable pearl relates to follow-up appointments for an evaluation of treatment. Suppose you are caring for a patient who has uncontrolled diabetes, and you start insulin. Let's say you have the patient return in a week for assessment, and during the return visit, you ask if the prescribed insulin is being taken. If the patient replies with a simple, "Yes," they are generalizing. A better way to clarify treatment is to ask, "How much insulin are you taking?" I can assure you the compliant patients know the answer without hesitation.

If the patient is taking basal-bolus insulin, ask, "How much of both are you taking and describe what the pen looks like by color." It is surprising how often patients can get confused when taking basal-bolus insulin, accidentally swapping the long-acting form for the short-acting form and vice versa. Make it simple for them. This can be confusing for even the smartest patients, especially when they're dealing with a new diagnosis. Also, realize that some patients may be afraid to let you know they are confused for fear of seeming dense, so I repeat, make it simple for your patients.

Gently pushing your patients to regurgitate what they are doing at home or what their values for BP and glucose are is the most compelling method of determining compliance to and effectiveness of treatment. Do not be fooled. Avoid the trap of generalizations.

11
Avoid Copying Work

As the provider, when caring for a patient in any setting, avoid copying other providers' work, regardless of how trivial it may seem to you. Please keep in mind that your notes are viewed over and over again. This point is especially true for hospital medicine APRNs.

Your colleagues, the physicians, and nurse practitioners are relying on you for accurate, authentic information. What you write immediately provides a picture of your understanding of the subject matter and confirms your knowledge, or lack thereof, of pathophysiology. Understand in detail what you are writing and be able to regurgitate anything you wrote in conversation with a physician or counterpart. Doing it this way is how trust and respect (mainly respect) are acquired. It would be a tragedy for you to copy another provider's work only to discover that their notes were inaccurate or lacked substance.

For example, as the hospitalist on a patient's case, I reviewed a note by the consulting infectious disease provider, which happened to be written by a colleague and nurse practitioner. I was not clear on what she wrote in the record regarding the patient's care, so I called her for clarification. She could not remember what she wrote, which in itself may not be alarming. However, what was alarming was when I read to her what was written, she explained that she was not sure what it meant and that another consultant wrote it, adding that she merely copied it forward.

The single most important thing nurse practitioners and providers must do in the field of medicine is be aware and precise. As NPs, we are critiqued more than anyone else in the profession, even more than the physician assistant. This is partially because the physician assistant is protected and governed by the physician. We must prove we know what we are talking about, and the only way to do that is to write what we know and question what does not make sense. What we do not understand should be investigated via research, which can be a quick Medscape or up-to-date inquiry. We live in an era where we have easy access to smartphones that grant us knowledge that is quite literally at our fingertips. It is imperative that we are informed, confident, and speak the language.

While mentioning the topic of speaking the language, I must inform you that medical provider lingo is moderately different from that of a nurse. These terms have often never been mentioned to nurses. For example, I once was reviewing a radiology report that mentioned "lingula pneumonia," and before that particular day, I had never seen the word "lingula" before. Upon further research, I learned that the lingula is the tongue-shaped region in the upper lobe of the lung. Physicians know this and easily understand this language directly out of school, whereas a nurse practitioner needs to spend time learning these little tidbits. Another way to speak the language is to talk as a provider and not a nurse (not that anything is wrong with nursing language). If you have graduated to the role of the provider, you must know how to articulate effectively with your peers (physicians, physician assistants, and other APRNs).

Simply paying attention and reading the notes of providers who exemplify what you want to become is a great way to pick up on certain terms. If a patient tells you, "I'm vomiting every time I cough," the way to state this as a provider is by saying the patient is experiencing "post tussive emesis."

The best way to get acclimated to the world of the provider is to stay attentive, consult often, engage in conversation with physicians and veteran conscientious NPs, and take the time to investigate and learn. School did not end when you graduated; it just began. Now, it is at your own pace and motivation level. If these criteria are met, you can stand out as a prudent nurse practitioner and can always be marketable, regardless of the potential market saturation.

12

ENGAGING WITH YOUR PHYSICIAN COLLEAGUES

I spoke briefly in the previous chapter about knowing the lingo and getting acclimated with talking with your peer physicians. I will briefly reiterate that you should know the lingo and further speak on what you should be prepared to know when speaking to a physician, NP, or provider. When speaking with a physician (especially a consult or referring physician) to gain more knowledge about an area you may not fully understand, always have a foundation or working knowledge of what it is you are speaking of. Simply put, do not talk blindly. The saying "No one is aware of a person's ignorance until they open their mouth" definitely rings true as it relates to ill-prepared conversations.

Always have a working knowledge of what you are inquiring about with a physician. I cannot stress this enough. While it is true that no one knows everything, always remember that your conversations with the physician or specialty NP groups are also interviews for the other party. Even if you do not have all the answers, the other provider will undoubtedly want to know that you can think your way through a situation or problem with pathophysiology. Once it is established that you have critical thinking skills and can bring forth some interpretation of what you have discovered about the issue at hand, you have passed the tests and are deserving of their knowledge. A physician or other provider will grow tired and lose respect for the provider who is always asking for knowledge in a leeching fashion but never takes the time to self-educate. Doing that is the easiest way to lose credibility with the physician or counter providers.

13
ACCEPT THE CHALLENGE

This topic goes right along with the theme of the previous chapter: Never, ever run from a challenge. Remember, your most significant battles are your most rewarding accomplishments. If a topic or patient appears complex to you, do not shy away. Do your homework. Trust the process. You are equipped to handle this. Your biggest asset is your brain. Remember, you are growing in the midst of the most uncomfortable situations.

When I was a novel APRN, what always kept me safe and prudent was keeping in mind what I did not know. Utilize your resources, and do not be afraid to ask intellectual questions. You will not know everything, but your questions should be initiated with what you do know. For example, you may not know why a patient has hyponatremia, but you should investigate why they have developed it. Depending on the patient's situation and state, it would be best to first review all possibilities before seeking the assistance of your collaborator, nephrologist, or neurologist. When requesting assistance, make sure you list what you have done prior to coming to them. Still using the given scenario, you can say, "I have evaluated medications, urine sodium, cortisol levels, glucose levels, and intake and output; however, I'm not convinced regarding the etiology. Are you able to look over my workup and give input regarding etiology?"

Break down every area of confusion. Just as nursing is a building block, so is the role of the provider. Start with the basics and build. An old nursing instructor of mine used to always tell the class, "Even if you do not know what it is, you better know what it is not." That statement still holds up today. You must have a working knowledge of what is considered normal to be able to quickly identify the abnormal because that will be the basis of what drives your workup. Medscape and Epocrates have exceptionally reliable resources for calculators, scoring tools like CHADS and TIMI, adjustment of calcium, dosage goals, and weight.

Anything you have not written or performed before should be investigated by one of these two resources prior to writing for a patient. Never be afraid to look up unfamiliar subject matter.

14

REMAINING CALM AND CONFIDENT (EVEN IF YOU DO NOT FEEL CONFIDENT INTERNALLY)

This chapter covers one of the most important topics for the novel APRN. As providers fresh out of school, we do not think of how hard the transition to a new role can be. Because we were such strong nurses and knew what the patient needed when calling the physician in our previous roles, we think the new role of provider is not going to be a big transition; however, this is simply not the case! *All* new roles are challenging, and you are not expected to be perfect. There will be plenty of new strategies, protocols, documentation, time management changes, and mental processing that were not present (to this degree) in most nurses' previous roles.

Feeling apprehensive, doubtful, useless, or possibly ill-prepared is *normal* as a novel APRN, so keep your feet planted forward and keep your head high. Also, do not be afraid to look up anything unfamiliar because that will help you learn and retain so many things that will be beneficial later. Consult and refer as much as you can (be careful about not researching and initiating workups before referral). It would be best to do your own research and workup prior to any consults or specialty referral placement. The specialist's job is not to do your work for you but, rather, to assist you and pick up after the basic identifying workup is performed. FYI: Specialists will screen referrals to see why you are consulting. They do not mind helping, but they, too, are extremely busy and prefer not to do the workup of the primary care provider.

Let's say a patient comes into your clinic with a chief complaint of right knee pain after falling. You examine the knee but do not find anything readily identifiable as abnormal. It is unacceptable for a provider to send that patient to an orthopedist for further evaluation without imaging and confirmation that there is, in fact, something for the orthopedist to intervene on.

Another good, and quite common, example are patients with polyarticular joint pain. Let's say you intuitively suspect the patient has rheumatoid arthritis. Although you may have postulated about the cause of what the patient is complaining about, it is unacceptable to refer the patient to a rheumatologist without doing the homework of ruling out all arthritic and autoimmune processes. In this case, the provider should obtain a detailed interview of symptoms, examine the patient, and get imaging if necessary. The next thing to do would be to send the patient for serologic testing to rule out rheumatoid arthritis, gouty arthritis, Systemic Lupus Erythematosus (SLE), and polymyalgia rheumatica (PMR). Upon completing serologic testing and receiving the results, the next step would be to refer the patient appropriately.

Never use physicians as your residents. They will become annoyed, possibly refuse your referrals, or perhaps treat your patients with the notion that you are too lazy to do so yourself. Some may even speak negatively of you to your patients. It is a crazy world. Respect is everything. If you form respect with them, you can send them anything with proper workup, and they will recognize it. They will call you for colleague-to-colleague conversations. Remember, your name is everything, and it is what will later determine your marketability for growth.

After consulting with your specialty physician and nurse practitioners, read and watch what they do, as it is primarily a learning tool for you. Do not just take what they are doing at face value. *Look it up!* Learn about what they are doing. You may need to emulate what you have now come to understand if you get a patient with inadequate resources and no access to specialties. Soak up all the information you can. Knowledge is a power that can never be taken from you. If you think you have found power as a provider, try backing it up with the most substantial knowledge base and lingo you can empower yourself with. You will be the talk of the establishment, a gem. Despite what you have to spend time learning, please be assured your university has taught you all you need to know for future skill-building. The APRN role is just like a nurse's role in the sense that it is a building block.

You are prepared. You are ready. Trust yourself and the process. Persevere through the uncomfortable because it is truly where you will grow. Keep your head up. No matter how nervous you are or how you feel talking to a patient for the first time, keep in mind that you are exactly where you should be in the process. Stay calm, try not to stutter or show nervousness, and learn as much about your patients before entering their presence so they can feel confident in your ability to care for them. You may be shaking in your boots, so to speak, but *never* let the patient see it. Remain calm. When you are nervous, the patient will become nervous and may begin to think 1) they are dying—so try not to be dramatic no matter what you see or how it surprises you—or 2) you are not qualified to care for them. You determine what box they put you in.

Patients come to us very vulnerable and frequently disclose information so sensitive to them that even their closest companion is oblivious. This is because of the level of trust they desire to establish with you. They hope you can fix what they are so nervous about. Sometimes they may feel you are their only hope. Imagine what a nervous, unconfident provider looks like to them. Now, I am not saying you cannot be nervous at all. There is a tremendous responsibility in this role, so of course, you are going to be nervous, but do not show it. Listen to your patients, think through what they are saying, go back and ask questions you may have forgotten, but maintain your cool. Exhale away from the patient, perhaps in your office or documenting room.

Upon graduation and certification, I was blessed enough to obtain a role as an advanced practice provider of a well-respected magnet hospital's hospital medicine department. However, I trained from an educational perspective in family medicine—big difference. My well-known, reputable school did not allow any hospital rotations during clinical phases. Upon obtaining this job, I was expected to complete a full detailed history and physical with a comprehensive assessment and plan of care within fifteen to twenty minutes per patient. This task was something I had upwards of three days to turn around when I was in school.

So I started my new role and interviewed the patient at the bedside. As I listened, more nervous than a preschooler on the first day of school, I thought to myself, *What am I supposed to do with what he is telling me?* I was lost.

I was a keen student, but I initially believed I was not prepared for the challenge. Keep in mind I never gave the impression of nervousness. I could only see four people in ten hours (no lie). Every day, I went home feeling low and useless, but I prayed and took the time to look everything up so I could use each experience and new piece of knowledge to my benefit in hopes of retaining it for my next encounter. I did the research, consulted workups, read consult notes, asked intellectual questions upon reading consult notes, and did more research. I did this every day for months, and I carried forward every day.

I remember being so angry when I walked into the hospital with five new admits and eight other patients to see plus discharges. I easily stayed sixteen hours some days just to finish my work (this was not mandatory, but I could not put it down). Every day for as long as I can remember (maybe three to six months), I drove home on the verge of crying, thinking I should quit. And in my most uncomfortable time, I was growing and molding into what I consider to be a strong prudent APRN.

I tell this story to say please do not give up when you are uncomfortable; this is when you are blossoming. You must feel uncomfortable to grow. If you are not uncomfortable, you are probably not learning to your maximum potential. Trust yourself, the process, and your foundation. You are ready!

15
KEEP GOD FIRST

In writing this book, I have primarily spoken from my heart on things the novel APRN may not know based on my personal experiences and the experiences of my colleagues. All the topics mentioned earlier are relatively crucial to your career as an APRN, but none, in my opinion, are as vital as this chapter. This chapter speaks on the center of your universe, God. Without Him, we would not be in the position we are in now.

The APRN's role encompasses a power and respect that most of us do not realize we have, especially the novel APRN. It is a proud moment when you start making decisions and understanding the effect you have on the patients and your peers. Be careful not to get caught up in the feeling and subconsciously (or consciously) create or exhibit feelings of superiority. Regardless of how powerful you feel in your new role, keep God first. He is the head *and* the tail. Nothing is given without His approval, and if abused, it will be taken away. I implore you to seek God daily before the start of your day. When you do this, you seek His protection from the things you cannot see, and you create a peacefulness in your spirit that the patient can feel.

As the new leader, you may not recognize how much you are being watched. How you are viewed is determined by your interactions with everyone, and your spirit heavily influences those interactions. The patients, nurses, doctors, housekeepers, certified nursing assistants, lab technicians, ward clerks, and family members, to name a few, are all observing you. They are observing your knowledge, kindness, empathy, humbleness, and general interactions. How you respond is grounded by pure love in God.

When we seek God daily before all else and allow Him to enter our spirit, we carry this special glow around with us. It is funny that we often hear preachers state, "This joy I have, man didn't give it, and man can't take it away." They are speaking of the calmness of your spirit when you know and trust God. I am sometimes surprised at the number of employees of all disciplines who walk up to me and tell me how proud they are of me and how they speak to their daughters in nursing school about me. This is humbling because you do not realize how many people are observing you.

I'll sum this chapter up with one verse from the Bible. In Matthew 6:33, Jesus himself stated, "But seek ye first the kingdom of God and His righteousness, and all these things shall be added unto you." God's word does not return void. Never, ever. If you seek God and keep Him first, the one thing I can surely promise you is success in your career and personal life. Be blessed and enter your new career doing God's will. May God bless all your endeavors.

Hopefully, this book has highlighted some of the necessary knowledge you must have to make an informed decision as it relates to your career. Please be mindful of your state regulations and utilize some of this advice to your advantage. I cannot wait to get your feedback regarding your experiences and salaries and how this book affected your decision-making and interactions. Talk to me. Tell me how these examples helped you.

Peace, love, and blessings to you forever.

Feel free to provide feedback about this book on my webpage: www. NPSENSE.com.

ABOUT THE AUTHOR

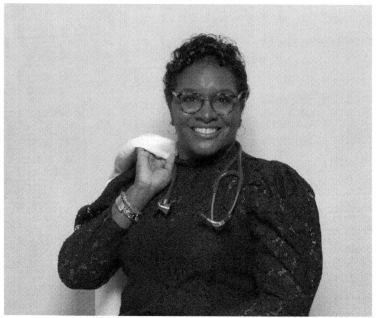

Shelita S. Carr is a nurse practitioner actively practicing in Chalmette, Louisiana. For the last seven years, she has been a nurse practitioner and graduated in 2013 from Loyola University of New Orleans with a concentration in family medicine. The bulk of her advanced practice experience has been in hospital medicine (since 2013), with the addition of clinic medicine starting in 2016. Since 2016, she has continued to practice both hospital and clinic medicine as an advanced practice registered nurse.

Mrs. Carr is married and empty-nesting with five adult progenies and four step-kids, all adulting and out of the home. Her passion is teaching, whether it is a patient, colleague, or nurse. Via her own words, "I am amazed by the human body, how it functions, and the continual state of learning this career has afforded me. My ultimate goal is to retire teaching, whether owning my own nursing school or virtual teaching via seminars, webinars, and private coaching."

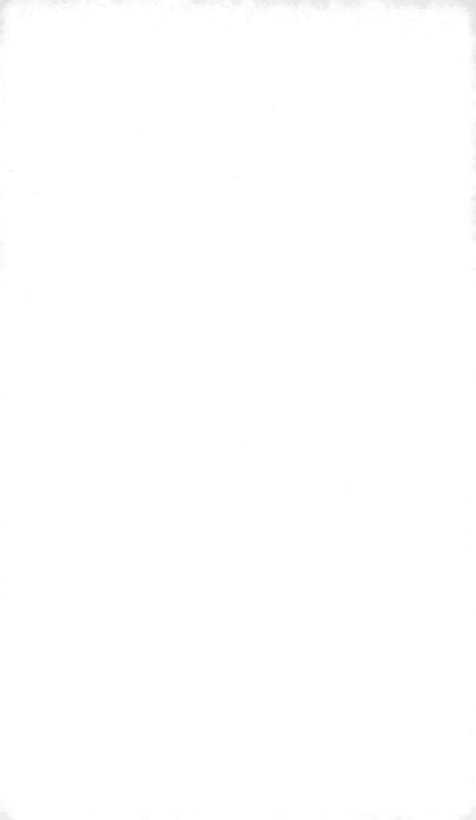

Made in the USA
Middletown, DE
18 April 2021

37849928R00054